I0468667

How to Become a Nurse

The Exact Roadmap That Will Lead You to a
Successful Career in Nursing!

Chase Hassen

Nurse Superhero

© 2015

Disclaimer:

Although the author and publisher have made every effort to ensure that the information in this book was correct at press time, the author and publisher do not assume and hereby disclaim any liability to any party for any loss, damage, or disruption caused by errors or omissions, whether such errors or omissions result from negligence, accident, or any other cause.

This book is not intended as a substitute for the medical advice of physicians. The reader should regularly consult a physician in matters relating to his/her health and particularly with respect to any symptoms that may require diagnosis or medical attention.

Have you seen my other NCLEX Prep Books?

NCLEX: Respiratory System : 105 Nursing Practice Questions and Rationales to Easily Crush the NCLEX!

NCLEX: Endocrine System : 105 Nursing Practice Questions and Rationales to EASILY Crush the NCLEX!

NCLEX: Cardiovascular System : 105 Nursing Practice and Rationales to Easily Crush the NCLEX!

NCLEX: Emergency Nursing : 105 Practice Questions and Rationales to Easily Crush the NCLEX!

EKG Interpretation: 24 Hours or Less to Easily Pass the ECG Portion of the NCLEX!

Lab Values: 137 Values You Know to Easily Pass The NCLEX!

First, I want to give you this FREE gift...

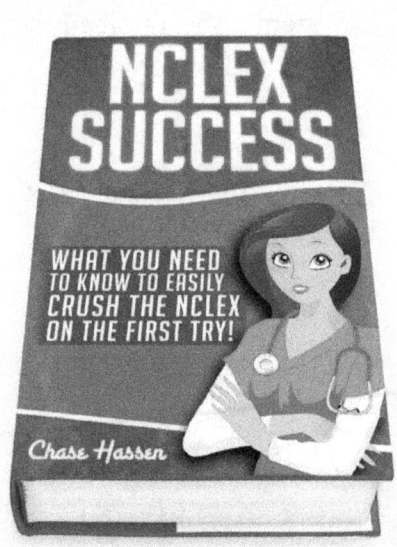

Just to say thanks for downloading my book, I wanted to give you another resource to help you absolutely crush the NCLEX Exam.

For a limited time, you can download this book for FREE.

http://bit.ly/1VNGAZ9

Table of Contents

Introduction

Being a nurse is an exciting job. If you like caring for patients as part of a dynamic and resourceful team, nursing might just be the career for you. Outside of patient care, there are opportunities for research, teaching, healthcare management and advanced practice nursing—if you know the right path to take.

There are several ways to become a nurse and many different types of nurses you can be. Knowing the pathways to becoming a nurse can help you take the required coursework without wasting time on the wrong classes. In this book, we will talk about the various pathways to nursing, including how to become a licensed practical nurse, registered nurse and an advanced practice nurse. You will understand how many years it takes to get the required coursework and what kind of career you will have once you take the classes and pass the national or state exams.

We will also talk about things you can do to increase your odds of getting into a good nursing school as well as getting a great job once you graduate. The nursing field is very competitive and you need to show through your actions and commitment to the medical field that you are both qualified and interested in the field of nursing. Good luck on your journey toward becoming a nurse!

Chapter 1:
Showing a Commitment

Nursing can be competitive so you need to do more than just get good grades in nursing school. Those who ultimately hire you will want to know if you have had any extracurricular activities in the area of nursing. There are various ways you can show this commitment. For example, you can take a two-three month course to become a Certified Nursing Assistant (CNA) prior to getting you nursing degree. CNAs work in home care, nursing home's and some hospitals, and are responsible for helping patients with their activities of daily living, including feeding, toileting and getting dressed by themselves (or with assistance). There is a need for nursing assistants in the field of nursing and you can work full or part time while getting your two or four year degree.

CNAs have a very difficult job to do but they play a large and helpful role in the care of patients. They make in the range of $10-$12 per hour, helping patients in a nursing facility or home care program to do things like the following:

- Positioning the patient in bed to prevent bed sores and increase joint mobility
- Feeding patients who need assistance in getting fed
- Grooming patients, such as bathing, hair washing, toenail and fingernail clipping, hair combing and tooth brushing or denture care.
- Assisting patients in ambulation or wheel chair use.

- Observe the patient's overall condition and measure things like food intake and liquid intake (along with output of urine and stool).
- Assist nurses in caring for patients under direct nursing supervision.
- Helping patients get in and out of bed.
- Getting the patient to the bathroom, commode or bed pan, depending on their abilities.

You can also do volunteer work at a hospital or nursing facility. Some hospitals have really good volunteer programs in which you can do things like getting a patient's water, providing books and other forms of entertainment for patients, and reading to them. Volunteering is something you can do in your spare time that is fun and helps you understand what it's like to be in a hospital or nursing home. Nursing schools will look positively on this kind of selfless commitment to patient care.

You can volunteer at community programs, such as health fairs in the community or through a corporation. This might mean handing out pamphlets geared toward the prevention and treatment of illness or you can check blood sugars or blood pressures. These things are easy to learn and can be very helpful to others.

Anything you can do in the healthcare field before nursing school or during your training will be looked upon favorably by the nursing school and/or any job you later seek. For example, you can work as a front desk person at a medical clinic or get training in other areas of healthcare like phlebotomy, which takes only a few months to learn. You may be able to find a job in that field while taking your nursing courses. Medical assisting work can be done in a clinic to prepare you for an advanced degree in the nursing field.

Chapter 2:
Two Year Nursing Programs

Two year nursing programs are offered at many community colleges and at some vocational schools. In a two year program, you graduate with a degree as an Associate Nurse. Such programs are taken over a period of 21 months to 24 months. Some schools will take you without a prior college education, while others will require you to have college level coursework in anatomy, nutrition, microbiology and math before starting nursing. You may have to take some general coursework in communication, humanities, and social sciences along with nursing courses. You will take nursing courses online or at the school with clinical rotations taken in various medical settings toward the end of your program.

As an associate nurse, you may be able to work in any clinic or in hospital departments such as mental health, emergency medicine, and pediatrics, among others. After the two year program you can get a practical nursing degree after passing the NCLEX-PN licensing examination.

Becoming an LPN has its advantages. For one, it takes less time. An RN generally takes a four year degree (and passing the NCLEX-RN exam). There is job growth in the LPN field—an estimated 22 percent increase in need for LPNs by the year 2020. On the other hand, some states are passing initiatives that will require a four year Bachelor's degree for all nurses so you want to keep track of the trends in your state.

Becoming an LPN means you'll probably be a candidate for an entry-level nursing position. Hospitals and clinics are looking for nurses fresh out of school so they can train them on the job in outpatient or inpatient medicine. By hiring new grads, they can train them the way they want to without having to give them large salaries until the nurse has been employed there for several years.

As a 2 year LPN, you have the opportunity to continue on to receive your Bachelor of Science degree in nursing (BSN) by taking coursework online, nights or weekends, while earning a living as an LPN. If pay is important to you, you will likely want to continue your education to become a four year RN. The average LPN makes about $40,000 per year, compared to the average RN, who makes about $65,000 per year.

Overall, going for your LPN in a two year program and licensure as an LPN has its advantages because you can quickly join the work force in a field of nursing that is currently undergoing a high rate of growth with the opportunity to study to become a four year RN as you continue on in your healthcare career.

You can sit for the NCLEX-RN program after taking a two year nursing degree as an associate nurse. If you pass the examination, you can work as a two year RN without spending so much money on tuition. It will be easier and faster to pay off your student loans after going through a two year program as opposed to a four year program. You can do basically the same job as a four year-trained RN but without all the tuition to pay back.

An obvious disadvantage to having a two year nursing degree (Associate's degree) is that you may be limited when it comes to furthering your career. Some areas of medical nursing require that you have your Bachelor's degree in Nursing (BSN) in order to work for them. While you can go through an LPN to RN program in a couple of years, there tends to be more things to juggle when you are older, such as school, work, children and spouse—all of which will need your attention when you are trying to complete a BSN degree after having your Associate's degree.

Chapter 3:
Your BSN Degree

The vast majority of BSN degrees require four years of schooling past high school, after which you will get a Bachelor's degree from many different universities and colleges. You get a nicely rounded liberal arts education to go along with your education in nursing. Classwork and clinical rotations are required along with more theory-related classes in leadership, research and things like disease management. This degree is a great stepping off program for just about any position in nursing as well as advanced degree programs (Master's degree equivalents). Bachelor's degree nurses take the NCLEX-RN test and, once passed, they become four year RNs.

The biggest advantages to becoming a four year RN is that you can always continue your education to become an advanced degree nurse and, if you choose to work as a four year RN, your pay will be higher than a two year degree nurse. If you decide to go into nursing areas such as nursing forensics, public health, research, and case management, you will need a BSN degree. If you want to go into teaching nursing, you will also need a four year (or more) degree. Your opportunities at larger hospitals and university hospitals are far greater if you have your Bachelor's degree in nursing.

The biggest disadvantage to working a four year program is that you will spend more money on tuition and you will less likely to be in the workforce until you get the BSN degree unless you have decided to go from a two year program to a four year program while working as an LPN or two year RN. You will likely need to get your schooling through a university-based program, which has a higher tuition than a community college.

If you think you might want to go into nursing management or get an advanced degree as a nurse practitioner, nurse midwife, or nurse anesthetist, you will need a four year degree. It all depends on what you are thinking of doing in the field of nursing. Fortunately, there are several different pathways to getting your nursing degree. You can start on one path and, if you change your mind down the road, you can switch gears and pursue further education and licensure options.

Some nursing programs are more competitive than others. Some have long waiting lists and don't accept everyone that applies to the school, while others seem to be easier to get into. If you have good high school grades and a background as a CNA or have volunteered in a healthcare situation, you will have a better chance to get accepted to a highly acclaimed school.

If all you want to do as a nurse is to care for patients in a hospital or clinic, you might just want to take the two year program and study for the NCLEX-RN exam. Both the two year and four year programs allow for students to take the NCLEX-RN examination to become a registered nurse. The job description for an RN, regardless of the number of years studying for the test, is much the same no matter what underlying degree you have.

Chapter 4:
The RN to BSN Program

As mentioned, you can go from a two year to four year BSN degree while working as an RN part time or full time, depending on how much spare time you have. RN to BSN programs often add the following courses to get your BSN degree:

- Health assessment

- Professional roles and values

- Evidence-Based Medicine

- Applied Nursing Research

- Care of the Elderly

- Nutrition for all ages of patients

- Organizational Systems

- Leadership in Nursing

- Application of Technology to Nursing

These courses prepare you for a greater leadership position in the field of nursing along with a higher salary. You may have more responsibilities when it comes to nursing management when you go from an RN to a BSN degree. Core courses, such as mathematics, anatomy and physiology, sociology, psychology, microbiology, biochemistry and statistics (among others) are usually transferrable from your two year program so you won't have to take them as part of your RN to BSN degree program.

Another advantage of getting your RN to BSN degree is that some healthcare facilities or hospitals will pay for your education while you work full time as an RN in their facility. This translates to free tuition and a great way to advance your career.

Both the RN and BSN programs have great future job expectations. It all depends on how much you want to put into your education and where you ultimately want to end up when it comes to your end-point in nursing. If all you want to do is care for patients in a hospital or clinic, the RN to BSN program may not yield anything more than a moderate increase in salary.

As a BSN, you will garner more respect from doctors and other healthcare professionals, who will know that you have more education than a two year degree. You will work with other professionals side-by-side and may have more opportunities for leadership in whatever field of nursing you choose to work in.

Chapter 5:
The NCLEX Examination

The term, NCLEX, stands for National Council Licensure Examination. This is the licensing tests all nurses must take in the US and Canada before becoming an LPN or an RN. There are two main NCLEX examinations: the NCLEX-RN for RNs and the NCLEX-PN for LPNs. Getting the license allows you to practice nursing as an RN or LPN. The NCLEX examination is run by the National Council of State Boards of Nursing, also known as the NCSBN. The test, once passed, means that you have met the requirements to practice in the field of nursing at the entry-level. The actual permission to work is dependent upon the state even though the NCLEX exam is a national examination.

Rather than your average paper and pencil test, the NCLEX exam is a computerized adaptive test or CAT format. The computer selects which question you must answer based on what you answered on the question before it. There is a lot of information and types of questions on the NCLEX test; the test is changed about every three years. The test questions are based on five key areas of nursing: analysis, assessment, intervention, planning, evaluation, and implementation.

If you take the NCLEX-PN examination, you will become a licensed practical nurse (LPN) or what's called a licensed vocational nurse (LVN). The test is on various aspects of nursing such as psychosocial integrity, health promotion, health maintenance, safe and effective care environment, infection control, physiological integrity, physiological adaptation, reduction of risk potential and pharmacological therapy.

The NCLEX-RN is taken to become a registered nurse. It covers some of the same areas as the NCLEX-PN examination with questions in the fields of gerontology, pediatrics, surgical care, adult medical care, infections disease and other areas of medicine. Pediatric questions deal with things common to children, such as burns, fractures, child abuse, congenital anomalies, and infectious diseases of kids. You will answer questions regarding having a safe care environment, health promotion, health maintenance, psychosocial integrity, pregnancy and pregnancy complications, mental health issues, substance abuse, and crisis intervention.

Questions are mostly multiple choice although more recently, a wider variety of questions are asked, including multiple correct answers, fill in the blank and picture questions. There are questions that ask the correct order of things. There are three levels of questions ranging from basic to complex. Ninety-five percent of questions are level 2 and level 3 questions. The number of questions you have to answer varies from person to person. You can take between 75 and 265 questions of which only 60 of the first 75 questions count. You will not know which questions count and which are just "trial questions" so it is best to answer each question as if it is the real thing. If you get a lot of questions about a similar topic, it could mean that one or more of the questions was a trial question or that you have answered some questions wrong, necessitating more questions in the same area to assess your skills.

There is no minimum time limit to this examination but there is a maximum time limit of 6 hours. You must take a ten minute break at the 2.5 hour mark and an optional break following the four hour mark. You cannot compare your score to another test taker because the whole thing is computerized and you will be taking a different number and type of questions than the next person who takes the test. If you meet or exceed the standard, you pass the test. If you do not meet or exceed the test standard, you fail the test.

Chapter 6:
Advanced Practice Nursing

Once you get your BSN, you can take the NCLEX-RN examination and can go on to training at a Master's degree level to be trained as an advanced practice nurse. Advanced practice nurses have a great deal of autonomy when compared to regular RNs. Your role in a healthcare team as an advanced practice nurse is far more independent and involves more leadership than LPNs or RNs.

You can become a **Certified Nurse Anesthetist** or CRNA by taking part in an accredited program in nurse anesthetist training. At the end of your education, you will likely find work at a hospital or freestanding surgery center that has a need for a CRNA to help in surgery, keeping patients under general anesthesia, controlling pain and keeping track of the vitals and health status of the patient undergoing surgery.

CRNAs across the US give 34 million people anesthetics during procedures and surgery and have been doing this since 1956. They have a special role to play in rural America where there aren't anesthesiologists around. In such cases, they help relieve pain in obstetrical patients, patients undergoing surgery, trauma stabilization and pain management in acute and chronic pain. Research has recently shown that there is essentially no difference in the type and quality of anesthesia care given by CRNAs and anesthesiologists, who are doctors by trade.

A CRNA plays a crucial role in a medical team that includes anesthesiologists, podiatrists, dentists, surgeons and surgical nursing staff. The CRNA provides anesthesia in the same way as their physician counterparts. CRNAs are highly respected in the medical world and basically work autonomously. CRNAs practice in hospitals, surgery centers, OB/GYN units, plastic surgery offices and pain management facilities. You can work in the private sector or for the military.

In order to get your degree and certification/licensure to become a CRNA, you need the following education and test taking:

You need a BSN or similar Bachelor's degree in a healthcare field.

You need to pass the NCLEX-RN and be a registered nurse.

You need to work in a critical care setting as a registered nurse for a minimum of one year so that you get critical care and ventilator experience.

You need a Master's degree through an accredited nurse anesthetist program. There are approximately 115 programs available to you in the US. The program takes about 24 to 36 months to complete and depends on the coursework you need and the various programs.

There is a National Certification Examination for Certified Nurse Anesthetists that you must pass to become a CRNA.

Recertification is done every two years by documenting your anesthesia practice, maintaining current licensure in your state and completing 40 hours of qualifying continuing education during the prior two years.

As a Certified Nurse Anesthetist, you will make approximately $110,000 USD starting out and, with experience, you can make up to $200,000 USD. The average salary for a CRNA is about $160,000 USD per year.

Another advanced degree program is that of a **Certified Nurse Midwife**. This is a Master's degree program in which you learn how to handle patients from pre-conception, through their pregnancy, through childbirth and in the postpartum period. They also do routine gynecological care for women of reproductive age. Once you get your education, you pass a certifying examination to become a certified nurse midwife or CNM.

A skilled midwife can do much to reduce the high Cesarean section rate found when OB/GYNs do deliveries. They have techniques to facilitate a normal vaginal birth and are less likely to jump to a Cesarean section if the labor becomes prolonged. CNMs attend to approximately ten percent of all spontaneous vaginal deliveries in the US. Ninety-seven percent of all these deliveries take place in a hospital, while about 2 percent take place in a freestanding birth center. Some CNMs will do home births and 1 percent of all CNM-assisted deliveries take place in the home of the patient.

Only about 10 percent of all the work a CNM does involves actual labor and delivery. The rest is clinical work in prevention and treatment of GYN disorders, primary care, prenatal care and postpartum care. They collaborate with different types of physicians to provide care to women of all ages. They work alongside Certified Midwives (CMs), who are midwives who did not get their nursing degree in the beginning. Newborn care is also the job of the certified nurse midwife.

A Certified Nurse Midwife can work in a variety of clinical settings. These include private clinics, public health clinics, hospitals, homes of their clients, and freestanding birth centers. They can work independently, for OB/GYN practices, and for HMOs interested in rounding out their staff to include CNMs.

The work of a CNM can be difficult, involving long hours during the night and weekends because deliveries do not happen at a set schedule. The median salary of a Certified Nurse Midwife is about $95,000. This means that half of all nurse midwives make less than this amount and half make more than this amount. Your salary will depend on who you work for, how much you work, your geographical location, and your experience. Many salaried CNMs have good benefit packages including retirement and healthcare provisions.

As an advanced practice nurse, you can become a Certified Nurse Practitioner (NP). This is also a Master's degree program in which you learn how to independently care for patients under the guidance of a physician. You can take care of anything from infants to the elderly and can work in a variety of specialties and settings. You can be a pediatric nurse practitioner, geriatric nurse practitioner, family nurse practitioner or psychiatric nurse practitioner, among others.

The scope of care provided by a nurse practitioner is varied and can include the management of many different diseases, including hypertension, immunization care, diabetes, injuries, mental health conditions and other common diseases. You will learn how to interpret EKGs, X-rays and laboratory tests. Most nurse practitioners prescribe medications independently of doctors, including DEA scheduled medications. Whether or not you can practice completely independently depends on the state you live in. Only about half the states allow you to practice independently.

As a nurse practitioner, you can work for HMOs, clinics, hospitals, community health centers, and as teachers of nurses. You can work in schools or for corporations and the military. About fifteen percent of all nurse practitioners thrive in their own private practice. You may work a 9 to 5 job during the week or all through the week, day or night, depending on where you work and your job description.

The median salary for a nurse practitioner is about $98,000. This means that half will earn less than that and half will earn more than that. The amount you earn depends on your experience, the geographical area you work in, how much you work, and the area of medicine you work in.

A CNS is a **Clinical Nurse Specialist** who has an advanced (Master's or Doctoral) degree a specific area of medicine. You may work for clinics that specialize in women's health, geriatrics or pediatrics. You can work in emergency departments, clinics or in critical care areas of the hospital. You can specialize in cancer care or diabetes, or work in rehabilitation or in mental health. What it means is that you have taken the time and effort to focus on a specific area of medicine that you subsequently work in. You can work as expert consultants for lower level nurses, such as RNs and LPNs or work in clinical care.

The salary of a Clinical Nurse Specialist is in the range of $50,000 USD to more than $100,000 USD. It all depends on the clinical specialty chosen by the CNS, experience, and where geographically you work.

Chapter 7:
Doctoral Nursing

You can further your education to get a PhD in nursing. From there, you can teach at a university level in the area of nursing or practice in medical research. You can get your doctoral degree by attending a doctoral nursing program at a university full time or part time, while working as a nurse in the field of your choice. As a PhD in nursing and with a scientific background, such as in biology, chemistry or biochemistry, you can work on research projects and publish in major medical journals.

As a nursing researcher, you study different aspects of health, including preventative care and the treatment of illnesses. You work in the areas of improving overall health, such as healthcare outcomes in scientific studies related to prevention and illness management. You design various studies that interest you and carry them out with the collaboration of other doctoral nurses, scientists, doctors, and pharmaceutical companies. You may be paid by a university to teach and do research or you can apply for federal and non-federal grants which will pay your salary and fund your research. Once your research study has been completed, you will write up your findings and publish them in various medical, scientific, or nursing journals and other publications.

Often you will need to start your road toward becoming a nurse researcher by working in a laboratory as a research assistant, or as a clinical research monitor or data coordinator. As you gain experience and ideas come to you, you can apply for a grant to become a principal investigator on your very own research study. Some things you might do research on include the following:

Ways to improve a terminal patient's quality of life

Enhancing patient safety by preventing injuries or illnesses

End of life care

Ways to deliver healthcare that is more efficient and effective.

Ways to help those with chronic illnesses

As a doctoral level nurse researcher and/or teacher, you will work with other scientists working in medicine, nutrition, pharmacology and engineering, depending on the type of research you plan to do. You can do research that changes the face of medicine in the future.

As a nurse researcher with a doctoral degree, you can work in a university setting, for a pharmaceutical company, in a laboratory or other setting. You may work for a profit-oriented company or a nonprofit corporation. Generally, because you work based on grant money, you will work on one project, apply for another grant and then work on another project. This can be a scary proposition without what seems like steady income. Grants, however, are usually always available if the research topic you choose is relevant and the grant is well-written. You must gain the skills of grant-writing a part of your doctoral nursing training and you will learn how to write up journal and research articles as you go along. You might have to present the findings of your research at major medical conferences, depending on the level of interest in your research.

A nurse researcher or doctoral level teacher/instructor makes in the range of $95,000 per year. You can work in research and supplement that income by working in the field of university or college-level teaching, writing texts, doing speaking engagements, and consulting work for other entities.

Chapter 8:
Conclusion

Working in nursing can mean many things and the pathways to get where you want to be are varied. You might gradually work your way up from a certified nursing assistant while training to get your two year degree, after which you can become an RN or an LPN. You can work as a two year nurse while taking online or night classes (plus clinical rotations) in order to become a four year educated nurse with an RN (after passing the NCLEX-RN examination). After working in the field for a while, you might decide to get your Master's degree and work as a certified midwife, clinical nurse specialist, certified nurse midwife, or certified nurse anesthetist.

In whatever path you choose, you make increasing amounts of money, based on your past experience, who you work for, the degree of education and the geographical location you work in. Your education can take only months, such as becoming a certified nursing assistant or CNA, or several years, in which you can come away with a Master's degree or Doctoral degree in the field of nursing. Tuition varies, depending on what type of degree you want as well as on the caliber of school you go to. Financial aid in the form of scholarships and student loans are available to those who qualify and, because nurses make a good salary on average, you should be able to pay back the loans in the years following your graduation.

Nursing is one of the few programs in which there are many pathways to success. You have the opportunity to work in the field after only a few months of training so you can see on the job the various choices of job you might want to have in the future. Being a nurse means being a part of a large medical team caring for patients on all levels of care. If you already know where you want to be and are sure of your decision, you can just take the classes necessary to get you where you want to go. If you are not sure, take a few classes and become certified as an LPN or even a CNA so that you can experience what it is like to work as part of a healthcare team, deciding to pursue your education further down the road while making a living with the degree you already have.

I want to thank you for purchasing my book! I hope you really enjoyed it. If so, do you mind doing me a quick favor and writing a review on amazon? It would be greatly appreciated!

I hope you received a ton of value from this book. I'll talk to you soon and see you in the next book!

- Chase Hassen

Nurse Superhero

Highly Recommended Books for Success

1. NCLEX: Cardiovascular System : 105 Nursing Practice and Rationales to Easily Crush the NCLEX!

2. NCLEX: Emergency Nursing : 105 Practice Questions and Rationales to Easily Crush the NCLEX!

3. Lab Values: 137 Values You Know to Easily Pass The NCLEX!

4. EKG Interpretation: 24 Hours or Less to Easily Pass the ECG Portion of the NCLEX!

5. Fluid and Electrolytes: 24 Hours or Less to Absolutely Crush the NCLEX Exam!

6. Nursing Careers: Easily Choose What Nursing Career Will Make Your 12 Hour Shift a Blast!

7. Night Shift: 10 Survival Tips for Nurses to Get Through The Night!

8. <u>NCLEX: Endocrine System : 105 Nursing Practice Questions</u> <u>and Rationales to EASILY Crush the NCLEX!</u>

And **MUCH MUCH MORE**! Visit my amazon author page to see more at:

http://amzn.to/1HCtfSy

www.ingramcontent.com/pod-product-compliance
Lightning Source LLC
Chambersburg PA
CBHW070308190526
45169CB00004B/1543